Richard KAMBALE KEUKEU

Hematological and biochemical tests:

Richard KAMBALE KEUKEU

Hematological and biochemical tests:

What are the clinical interpretations?

ScienciaScripts

Imprint

Cover image: www.ingimage.com

This book is a translation from the original published under ISBN 978-613-8-45113-6.

Publisher:
Sciencia Scripts
is a trademark of
Dodo Books Indian Ocean Ltd. and OmniScriptum S.R.L publishing group

120 High Road, East Finchley, London, N2 9ED, United Kingdom
Str. Armeneasca 28/1, office 1, Chisinau MD-2012, Republic of Moldova, Europe
Managing Directors: Ieva Konstantinova, Victoria Ursu
info@omniscriptum.com

Printed at: see last page
ISBN: 978-620-8-56293-9

Foreword

This document has been designed to help medical students familiarize themselves with the various laboratory examinations, mainly those relating to haematology and biochemistry.

Indeed, the main aim of this future practitioner, the medical student, is to save human lives.
Clinical laboratories enable doctors to make precise diagnoses, and also to monitor their patients, either for check-ups or during epidemics. All this contributes to improving quality of life.

In view of the above, we understand why it is so urgent for this future doctor to be sufficiently equipped to interpret the results of these laboratory tests for better patient care.

Nevertheless, students often find it difficult to correlate these essential laboratory tests with clinical practice.

This concise and precise book addresses this deficiency by covering the hematology and biochemistry tests commonly requested in our field.
It therefore covers each test, specifying *its role, normal values and clinical relevance.*

Thanks

Our thanks go first and foremost to our God, who continues to grant us life and health.

Our most sincere and considerable thanks to the Ministry of Higher and University Education of the Democratic Republic of Congo for switching to the LMD system, which supports student research.

To the authorities of the Free University of the Great Lakes Countries in general, and to the heads of the Faculty of Medicine in particular, for the quality of training they offer us.

We'll always be grateful for all the efforts and sacrifices our parents KAMATE SIBUYAKULA Bonne-année and BAHANI HANGI Brigitte have made on our behalf.

To those who have supported us from near and far, we reiterate our gratitude.

Table of contents

Foreword

With the aim of contributing to the learning of haematology in general and clinical biology in particular, we medical students have had the courage to write this few-page book containing a minimum of information on routine haematological and biochemical examinations and their clinical interpretations.

Indeed, in the student world, correlating the results of paraclinical examinations with the clinic poses a serious problem, because it requires practical experience on the part of the learner.

That's why we'd like to take this opportunity to help medical students in our area master the clinical translation of haematological and biochemical tests commonly requested in our health facilities.

Part I: HEMATOLOGY

1. Red blood cells or erythrocytes or red blood cells

They are round cells, filled with hemoglobin. Viewed from the side, a red blood cell looks like a disk, thinned at the center, and contains no nucleus. Red blood cells carry hemoglobin, which combines with oxygen to transport it from the lungs to the tissues.

- ***Normal values :***

Me	4.5 to 6.2 x 10^6/mm^3
Femal	4 to 5.4 x 10^6/mm^3
Child (1 year	3.6 to 5 x 10^6/mm^3
Newbor	5 to 6 x 10^6/mm$^{(3}$

2. Hemoglobin

Hemoglobin, which gives blood its red color, is a protein that binds, transports and delivers the oxygen essential for life.

It is made up of two linked α-globins and two β-globins, each containing an iron-containing "heme".

- ***Normal values***

Men	13 to 18 g/dL.
Female	12 to 16 g/dL.
Pregnant woman (early ^{2nd} trimester): 10.5 to 14 g/dL.	
Children over 2 years: 12 to 16 g/dL.	
Newborn: 14 to 20 g/dL.	

- ***Clinical interpretation***

- ❖ When the hemoglobin value is below the normal range, we speak of ***anemia***.

  It requires rapid assessment of tolerance (*cardiac insufficiency, hypovolemic shock*) and elimination of rapidly evolving diagnoses (*haemorrhage, malaria, etc.*) in order to rapidly start symptomatic and etiological treatment.
- ❖ When the hemoglobin value is higher than the normal range, we speak of ***polyglobulia***.

3. Erythrocyte constants

Red blood cell count, hemoglobin level and hematocrit are used to calculate globular indices or erythrocyte constants.

These are *mean corpuscular volume (MCV), mean corpuscular hemoglobin concentration (MCHC) and mean corpuscular hemoglobin content (MCHC).*

- ***Normal values***

- **VGM** = hematocrit/red blood cell count

  It is expressed in femtoliter (fL). It varies between **85 and 98** fL in adults.
- **The mean corpuscular haemoglobin concentration** (MCHC) expresses, in g/dL (or %), the mean haemoglobin concentration of red blood cells (MCHC Hb) = haemoglobin/haematocrit.

  It varies between **32 and 36g/l**

- The mean corpuscular hemoglobin content (MCHC) expresses in pg/cell), the quantity of hemoglobin contained in a red blood cell: MCHC Hb = hemoglobin/number of red blood cells.

  It varies between **27 and 32 pg/cell** in adults.

- ***Clinical benefits of erythrocyte constants***

✓ In adults, a GMV below 85 fL defines ***microcytosis***, and a GMV above 95 fL ***macrocytosis***.

✓ An HACC below 32 g/dL indicates ***hypochromia***, and an HACC between 32 and 36 g/dL ***normochromia*** (no hyperchromia).

✓ Less widely used than HSMT, HSMT is more sensitive than HSMT for judging ***hypochromia***.

4. White blood cells or leukocytes

- ***Normal values***

GB (L/L)	4-10 G/L
Neutrophils	1.5 to 7 G/L
Eosinophils	< 0.5 G/L
Basophils	< 0.05 G/L
Lymphocytes	1 to 4 G/L
Monocytes	0.1 to 1 G/L

- ***Clinical benefits***

✓ **Neutrophilic polymorphism (WBC > 7,000/mm3)**

Polynucleosis is physiological during pregnancy, or induced by stress, physical exertion, surgery or corticosteroid therapy.
Classically, polynucleosis is associated *with bacterial infection or hepatic amebiasis.*

✓ **Neutropenia (WBC < 1,500/mm3)**

Excessive margination is a priori without infectious risk (PNN stuck to the surface of vessels without altering their functionality) in subjects of African origin, and can be unmasked by exercise. The main etiologies *of acute neutropenia are viral and iatrogenic.*

✓ **Hyper**

It points us in *the* direction of *parasitic infections, mainly helminths* (ascariasis, hookworm, anguillosis, trichinosis, bilharziosis, toxocariasis, filariasis), as well as certain allergies and other conditions.

✓ **Hyperlymphocytosis (L > 4,000/mm3)**

Hyperlymphocytosis is common *in viruses and trypanosomiasis*. It is sometimes associated with lymphoid hemopathy.

✓ **Lymphopenia (L < 500/mm3)**

Lymphopenia is usually observed in the course of *viruses (especially HIV infection) and hematological diseases.*

✓ **Monocytosis**

It points to *virosis, malaria, trypanosomiasis, syphilis, rickettsiosis, brucellosis and tuberculosis.*

5. Blood platelets

They play an important role in blood coagulation.

- ***Normal value:*** **150-400,000 per mm3 of blood**

- ***Clinical benefits***

✓ **Thrombocytopenia (platelets < 150 G/L)**

Any thrombocytopenia without signs of bleeding should be checked on an EDTA tube for false thrombocytopenia due to aggregation, which is usually reported by the laboratory.
The most thrombopenic infections are *malaria and viral infections (arboviruses, HIV).*
More rarely, *leptospirosis, borreliosis, rickettsiosis, babesiosis or disseminated histoplasmosis* may be evoked.
Severe sepsis can lead to disseminated intra-vascular coagulation.
Thrombocytopenia is also *an integral part of two serious bleeding syndromes, DIC and TTP* (thrombotic thrombocytopenic purpura or Moskowitz disease).

✓ **Thrombocytosis (platelets > 450 G/L)**

Classically, moderate thrombocytosis is observed *during pregnancy, martial deficiency, chronic hemolysis, and in the aftermath of splenectomy or asplenism.*

More rarely, it is the sign of a hemopathy, the most common of which *is essential thrombocythemia.*

Thrombocytosis > 1000 G/L is a risk factor for thrombotic events, requiring appropriate treatment and long-term prevention with salicylates.

6. Reticulocytes

Reticulocytes are red blood cells that have been in circulation for less than 48 hours. They can be recognized by a special staining that highlights the reticulum (reticulocytes) they contain, made up of ribosomal remnants. They are counted by most automated systems.

- ***Normal value:*** ***25 to 100 G/L***
- ***benefits***

Reticulocytosis, which reflects the medullary production of red blood cells in the last 48 hours, distinguishes :

- regenerative anemias where reticulocytosis is > 150 G/L and
- Aregenerative anemias.

7. Red cell sedimentation rate (VS)

Red blood cell sedimentation in a vertical tube (Westergren tube) is influenced by various factors, including the plasma concentration of proteins involved in inflammation and serum immunoglobulins.

- ***Normal value***

Normal value	**Men**	**Woman**
Young	Less than 15 mm	Less than 20 mm
Over 65	Less than 20 mm	Less than 25 mm

- ***Clinical benefits***

The SV is increased in inflammatory states, whatever the cause: *infectious or rheumatic diseases, connective tissue diseases, cancers, tissue necrosis*, etc.

In these cases, the acceleration of the SV correlates with an increase in "inflammation proteins" (haptoglobin, orosomucoid, etc.), with the exception of C-reactive protein.
It can also be elevated in cases of *chronic hepatitis, lupus, HIV infection, mixed cryoglobulinemia, IgA-deposited glomerulonephritis, etc.*

SV is of little diagnostic significance, except perhaps in cases of Horton's temporal arteritis.

However, it is standard practice to look for myeloma, Waldenström's disease and possibly B lymphoma when the SV exceeds 120 mm, *as monoclonal gammopathies are among the conditions with the highest SVs.*

8. Emmel's test

The Emmel test is used to screen for sickle cell hemoglobin S.

- ***Clinical relevance***: the test is positive in cases of sickle cell disease

9. Bleeding time or Duke's method

- ***Principle***

  A vaccinostyle is used to make a small incision incision is made in the earlobe. This wound bleeds and the time it takes for the bleeding to stop is measured.

- ***Normal value***: **2 to 4 minutes**

- ***clinical benefits***: why use this method?

This test is performed :

- for the diagnosis of certain haemorrhagic diseases,
- before surgery,
- before puncturing the liver or spleen.

10.Clotting time or Lee and White method

- ***Principle***

Venous blood is drawn into a glass tube. The time it takes to coagulate is measured. This test is of limited value, as it can only detect serious coagulation anomalies.

- ***Normal value:*** ***4 to 8 minutes***

- ***Clinical benefits***

A patient with an abnormally long coagulation time should be referred to a specialist for further examination.

11.Blood grouping

Why determine a patient's blood type?

The aim of a blood transfusion is to enable a patient to receive blood safely. This requires..:

- to determine the blood group or blood type of the patient,
- that his or her blood is carefully checked for compatibility with that of a suitable donor.

In the ABO system, it's the antigen found on the erythrocyte that determines the group, which is why :

- Group A (A antigen on the erythrocyte and anti-B antibodies in the serum) ;
- Group B (B antigen and anti-A antibodies) ;
- Group 0 (A and B antigens absent, but anti-A and anti-B antibodies) ;
- Group AB (A and B but neither anti-A nor anti-B).

In the Rhesus system, it is rather the presence of the D antigen in the plasma:

- Rhesus positive: presence of D antigens
- Rh-negative: absence of D antigens

Other systems

Li, Lutheran, P, Lewis, MN, Kidd, Kell, Duffy, etc. They are less important for the prevention of hemolytic birth defects or transfusion reactions.

12.Coumbs

The Coombs test is designed to detect antibodies attached to the surface of red blood cells and liable to cause immunological hemolysis.
These are usually *autoantibodies*.

Coumbs direct

The direct Coombs test (so called because it is performed in a single step) detects antibodies (immunoglobulins) attached to the surface of *red blood cells* by an agglutination reaction using human antiglobulins (*an anti-IgG antiglobulin and an anti-complement antiglobulin*).

The antibody can be titrated by making increasing dilutions of anti-immunoglobulin serum.
The test is increasingly performed by automated systems using agglutination techniques with gel or bead filtration.

Indirect Coumbs

The purpose of this test is to detect antierythrocyte antibodies in the patient's *serum*. It is performed in two stages.

❖ ***Clinical interest***

The Coombs test is used to identify "immunological" hemolytic anemias. "**immunological**" anemias, due to the presence of antibodies on the surface of red blood cells, causing their destruction.

We can have :

- Alloimmunization hemolytic anemias

Post-transfusion hemolysis is due to alloantibodies acquired following previous transfusions.

They are prevented by an indirect Coombs test. Hemolytic disease of the newborn is linked to immunization of a Rhesus-negative mother against Rhesus-positive fetal red blood cells.

- Autoimmune hemolytic anemias (AHAI)

The diagnosis of autoimmune hemolytic anemia is based on the positivity of a direct Coombs test, which proves the existence of an antibody on the surface of red blood cells and specifies its IgG or IgM class, with or without complement.

Part II: BIOCHEMISTRY

13.Microalbuminuria

The presence of low levels of albumin in urine, lower than the proteinuria detected by test strips (300 mg/24 h) but higher than physiological proteinuria (30 mg/24 h), is a marker of incipient nephropathy, particularly in diabetics and hypertensives.

- ***Normal value***: Microalbuminemia is defined as urinary albumin excretion of between ***30 and 300 mg/24 h or between 20 and 200 μg/min.***

- ***Clinical benefits***
  - ✓ in type 1 or type 2 diabetics, microalbuminuria raises the risk of *nephropathy* in the following 10 years (risk ×20);
  - ✓ in non-insulin-dependent type 2 diabetics, microalbuminuria is a *cardiovascular* risk factor;
  - ✓ in hypertensive patients, whether diabetic or not, microproteinuria is a risk factor for *coronary heart disease* (risk × 4).

14.Ketone compounds in urine

Normally, urine does not contain ketone bodies. However, acetone and other ketone compounds may appear in the urine, in which case the condition is known **as acetonuria**.

- ***Clinical benefits***

Acetonuria may be present :

- ✓ in certain types of severe or poorly controlled diabetes,
- ✓ in other conditions (dehydration, vomiting, malnutrition) or after violent exercise.

15.Glycorachy

This is the measurement of glucose in cerebrospinal fluid.

- ***Normal value***

In healthy individuals, the CSF glucose content is ***2.5 to 4.2 mmol/l*** (equivalent to 45 to 75 mg/100 ml in traditional units).

- ***Clinical benefits***

In cases *of meningitis* (especially *purulent meningitis*), the glucose content of the CSF is greatly reduced.

16.Albuminorachie

This is the determination of albumin in cerebrospinal fluid.

- ***Normal value***

Normal CSF protein content is **0.1 to 0.45 g/l.**

- ***Clinical benefits***

Albuminorachy increases with :

- ✓ meningitis, subarachnoid haemorrhage or
- ✓ spinal compression
- ✓ African trypanosomiasis.

17.Biliary pigments

The bile secreted by the liver contains greenish-yellow substances known as bile pigments.

- ***Interest***

In certain circumstances :

- ✓ liver disease (jaundice).
- ✓ anemias,
- ✓ infections ...

These pigments can pass into the bloodstream and then into the urine.

18.Rivalta

The Rivalta test is used to characterize the effusion fluid. A positive Rivalta test indicates a protein content in excess of **3 grams per 100 ml**, in which case the fluid is **exudative**.

A negative Rivalta test indicates a transudative, i.e. protein-free, fluid.

The Rivalta test is no longer used at laboratory level, mainly because the method has never been strictly standardized.

19.Blood glucose

This is the level of glucose in the blood. In normal subjects, blood glucose levels are kept stable, at around **5.5 mmol/L (fasting)**, by a complex neurohumoral system in which the insulin-glucagon pair plays an important role.

Diabetes mellitus is characterized by permanent hyperglycemia.

- ***Normal values***

➢ Fasting plasma glucose: 3.9 to 5.5 mmol/L.
➢ Postprandial glycemia (adult): < 7.8 mmol/L.
➢ Postprandial glycemia (pregnant women) : < 6.7 mmol/L.

Knowing that :

- g/L × 5.56 = mmol/L ;

- mmol/L × 0.18 = g/L.

- ***Clinical benefits***

➢ **Diabetes mellitus**

Hyperglycemia is the fundamental sign of diabetes mellitus. Blood glucose levels are above 2 g/L (11 mmol/L).

The diagnosis of diabetes is based on WHO criteria published in July 1998, defining *diabetes mellitus as fasting blood glucose ≥ 7 mmol/L (1.26 g/L), recorded on two occasions.*

Glycated hemoglobin testing used to be inadvisable for diagnosing diabetes. Today, glycated hemoglobin is considered to be less sensitive to the vagaries of fasting, which is required of patients before fasting blood glucose levels can be measured.

A distinction is made between **insulin-dependent or type 1 diabetes mellitus** (around 15% of diabetes cases) and **non-insulin-dependent type 2 diabetes** (around 85% of cases), depending on whether or not hyperglycemia is associated with ketosis and weight loss.

- **Hypoglycemi**

In adults, hypoglycemia is defined as a blood glucose level below **0.50 g/L (2.75 mmol/L)** on an empty stomach, or when feeling unwell.
Signs :

- ✓ headaches, concentration and speech problems
- ✓ diplopia, facial paresthesias ;
- ✓ sudden hypoglycemic coma with convulsions.

Hypoglycemia is sometimes secondary to :

- ✓ gastrectomy;
- ✓ adrenal or pituitary insufficiency;
- ✓ a thoracic or abdominal mesenchymal tumor;
- ✓ multiple liver metastases.

20.Gamma glytamyltransferase (Gamma GT)

This enzyme, found mainly in **the kidney and liver** but widespread throughout the body, catalyzes the first stage of **glutathione** degradation.

The enzyme circulating in plasma seems to be mainly of hepatic origin, since while its increase is frequent in hepatobiliary disorders, it is not observed in kidney diseases.

- ***Normal values***

Varies with assay techniques but is < **35 U/L**.

- ***Clinical benefits***

➢ **<u>Hepatobiliary disorders</u>**

Elevated gamma-GT is a good sign of *cholestasis*, whether intra- or extra-hepatic.

Cholestasis can be recognized by *the concomitant elevation of alkaline phosphatases.*

Gamma-GT is very high (>10×N) **in extra-hepatic biliary obstruction**, and elevated **in hepatocellular carcinoma and liver metastases**.

It is moderately elevated (< 10 × N) in *viral hepatitis and liver cirrhosis.*

➢ **<u>Medicines</u>**

Certain enzyme-inducing drugs (antidepressants, barbiturates, hydantoins, rifampin, etc.) increase gamma-GT (between 2 × N and 5 × N).

- **Alcoholism**

An increase in gamma-GT (above 2×N) is a good sign of alcoholism, not acute but chronic (more than 3 weeks), detecting nearly 70% of excessive drinkers (more than 80 g alcohol/day).

As a sign of alcoholism, gamma-GT elevation is not easy to interpret, as its specificity is very low.

- **Other**

Conditions as diverse as pancreatitis, myocardial infarction, certain brain tumors, epileptic seizures and thyroiditis can increase gamma-GT.

21. Transaminases (ALAT and ASAT)

Transaminases (or aminotransferases) are active in the liver, heart and muscles.

They pass into the serum in the event of **hepatic or muscular cytolysis.**

- ***Locations***

  - ✓ **Alanine aminotransferase** (ALAT, formerly GPT) is found mainly in the liver,
  - ✓ **aspartate aminotransferase** (ASAT, formerly GOT) in the heart.

- ***Normal values***

ALT: **5 to 35**
AST: **5 to 40 UI/L**

These values increase with weight (notify the laboratory in the event of obesity).

Clinical benefits

ALT increases more than AST in liver disease, and AST more than ALT in muscle necrosis.

Elevated transaminases are seen in *hepatic cytolysis and muscle necrosis.*

- **Hepatobiliary disorders**

- ***Acute elevations***

  A very significant increase in AST and especially ALT (N×10 to N×100) is observed in cytolysis **of viral, toxic, drug or liver hepatitis, shock (pulmonary embolism) or during intracholecular calculous migration**.

- ***Chronic elevations***

Chronic elevation of ALT to less than 3 times normal suggests :

- ✓ chronic alcoholism;
- ✓ chronic hepatitis C, where transaminases are often low;
- ✓ hepatic steatosis in obese patients or hypertriglyceridemic diabetics whose liver is "shiny" on ultrasound;
- ✓ certain medications: anti-epileptics, lipid-lowering drugs.

- **Cardiac disorders**

A very large increase (N×10 to 100) in ALT and especially ASAT is seen:

- ✓ in heart failure, where it reflects hypoxemic centrolobular hepatocyte destruction;
- ✓ in myocardial infarction, where its elevation occurs too late to be diagnostic;

✓ in muscular disorders such as myositis and myopathy.

Caution: To detect hepatic cytolysis, a single transaminase assay (preferably ALAT) is sufficient.

22.Blood urea

Blood urea is still required to detect *renal failure*, although this measurement is not very *sensitive*, as blood urea only exceeds normal limits when nephron levels are reduced by more than half.

- *Normal value*: **2.5 to 10 mmol/L (i.e. 0.10 to 0.50 g/L)**
- ***Clinical interest*** :

Elevated urea and creatinine go hand in hand *in organic renal failure.*

There is no need to request both a urea and creatinine test to detect renal failure.

23.Creatinine

It is a catabolite of muscle creatine, and is eliminated in the urine.

Reminder: We know that creatinine is eliminated by the kidney solely by filtration, and is neither reabsorbed nor secreted (or very little) by the tubule. There is a correlation between plasma creatinine concentration and glomerular filtration rate, in the sense that when glomerular flow rate falls, a higher concentration in the glomerular filtrate enables as much creatinine to be eliminated.

Plasma creatinine concentration depends neither on urine volume nor on diet.

- ***Normal values***

In men: 80 to 110 µmol/L (9 to 13 mg/L). In women: 60 to 90 µmol/L (7 to 10 mg/L). In children under 5: 20 to 40 µmol/L.
Note: During pregnancy, due to the physiological increase in renal blood flow, plasma creatinine falls below 50 µmol/L.

- ***Clinical benefits***
  - **Chronic renal failure**

As a reflection of glomerular filtration rate, creatinine levels can be used to monitor progress in chronic renal failure.

- **Acute renal failure**

The diagnosis of acute renal failure (ARF) is not based on diuresis criteria, as renal failure can be anuric (< 100 mL urine), oligoanuric (100 to 500 mL), or diuresis-preserved.
It is based on ***a rapid rise in creatinine, judged on two successive tests.***

24. Alkaline phosphatases

These membrane-bound enzymes are present in most of the body's tissues, but especially in **bone and liver**, where they are also eliminated via bile.

Alkaline phosphatase (ALP) is also measured to identify *liver or bone disorders*.

- ***Normal values***

✓ in adults: 50 to 130 IU/L ;

✓ in children: 100 to 200 IU/L.

Clinical benefits

❖ **Elevated alkaline phosphatases**

➢ ***Elevation of hepatic origin***

Elevated LAP is a good sign of **cholestasis**, whether **intra- or extrahepatic**. Cholestasis can be recognized by the concomitant elevation of gamma-GT (unlike bone diseases).

The most frequent intrahepatic cholestases are due to *viral or alcoholic hepatitis*.

Extrahepatic cholestasis is caused *by choledochal lithiasis and pancreatic cancer.*

➢ ***Elevation of bone origin***

In the absence of cholestasis, elevated PALs indicate increased **osteoblastic** activity, i.e. increased **osteoformation**:

- In children, **rickets** is the main cause.
- In adults, it is in **Paget's disease**

It is important in *osteomalacia due to vitamin D deficiency, hyperparathyroidism with bone lesions, and condensing bone metastases (prostate cancer)*.

❖ **Decrease in alkaline phosphatase**

A decrease in plasma alkaline phosphatase is only observed in the exceptional case of **hereditary hypophosphaturia (hypophosphatasia)**. It is an autosomal recessive disease, characterized by *rickets, early dental problems* (tooth loss as early as 20th years) and chondrocalcinosis.

25.Amylases

These are the *starch-hydrolyzing* enzymes produced by *the pancreas and salivary glands*

They are released into the serum whenever ductal obstruction or cell necrosis occurs in these glands, and then into the urine.

- ***Normal value***

In adults: **10 to 45 U/L** Note: Amylasemia is low at birth. Adult values are reached between 5 and 10 years of age.

- ***Clinical benefits***

➢ ***Salivary hyperamylasemia***

In mumps, bacterial infections, tumors or lithiasis of the salivary glands, a moderate rise in amylasemia is usual.

Chronic alcoholism also causes a modest increase (N×2 or N×3) in salivary amylasemia.

➢ ***Pancreatic hyperamylasemia and abdominal pain syndromes***

Hyperamylasemia is a good sign ***of acute pancreatitis***, *provided high concentrations (at least N×5) are required.*

➢ **<u>Other</u>**

Apart from pancreatitis, hyperamylasemia can be observed in a number of painful abdominal syndromes: calcific migration through the hepatopancreatic ampulla, ulcer perforation (passage of amylase-containing gastric fluid into the peritoneal cavity), mesenteric infarction, hemoperitoneum.
Retrograde wirsungography and opiate injections (Oddi spasm) can also increase amylasemia.

26.Uric acid

Uric acid is the end product of the breakdown of three purines (guanine, hypoxanthine and xanthine), a small proportion of which comes from the diet, and the majority from endogenous purinosynthesis resulting from the catabolism of nucleic acids.
It is eliminated in the urine.

+ *Normal values :*

Male: 40 to 60 mg/L or 240 to 360 µmol/L. Female: 30 to 50 mg/L or 180 to 300 µmol/L. Children: 25 to 40 mg/L or 150 to 240 µmol/L.

+ *Clinical benefits*

➢ **Hyperuricemia (> 70 mg/L or 416 µmol/L)**

- *Primary hyperuricemia, gout*

Most hyperuricemia is *primary* and indicative *of primary gout.*

- *Secondary hyperuricemia*

due to increased uric acid production, as in beer binges, or tumor lysis caused by chemotherapy of hematological malignancies (countered by infusion of recombinant urate oxidase).

- **Hypo-uricemia (< 25 mg/L or 150 µmol/L)**

There are three causes of hypo-uricemia:

- medication that inhibits uric acid synthesis (allopurinol) or increases its clearance (phenylbutazone), by far the most frequent case;
- reduced uric acid synthesis associated with severe liver failure, or hereditary xanthine oxidase deficiency (very rare);
- increased urinary uric acid excretion due to tubulopathy (Fanconi syndrome) or idiopathic causes.

27.Total albumin

Synthesized by the liver, albumin acts as a transporter for numerous ligands and plays a vital role in maintaining plasma oncotic pressure.

It is by far the most abundant protein in serum (60% of serum proteins).

- ***value***

In adults and children over one year of age: **40 to 50 g/L (650 to 800 µmol/L)**

- ***Clinical benefits***

- **Insufficient input or synthesis**

They may be due to insufficient amino acid intake (undernutrition): *hypoalbuminemia* is part of a polycardiac picture.

They are mainly caused by *hepatocellular insufficiency.*

- **Protein loss**

Nephrotic syndromes

Urinary losses of albumin characterize the nephrotic syndrome. Defined by albuminemia < 30 g/L and proteinuria > 3 g/day (50 mg/kg/day in children), a nephrotic syndrome is easy to recognize.

Malabsorptions

Digestive losses of albumin are due to malabsorption, usually discovered during the assessment of chronic diarrhea. All malabsorptions due to chronic enteropathies, celiac disease, Whipple's disease, short small bowel, intestinal lymphoma, can lead to hypoalbubinemia.

In adults, celiac disease is characterized by diarrhea, abdominal pain and, in 20% of cases, malabsorption with hypoalbubinemia, anemia and folate deficiency.

28.Creatine kinase (CK) or creatine phosphokinase (CPK)

Creatine kinase (CK) is widespread in *muscle, myocardium and brain.*

It is made up of two sub-units**,** **M** (*muscle*) and **B** (*brain*), which are at the origin of three iso-enzymes**:** **MM** (skeletal muscle), **BB** (brain), **MB** (myocardium).

- ***Normal values***

In adults: 15 to 150 IU/L CK levels are very high in newborns and remain elevated for up to a year.

- ***Clinical benefits***

➢ **<u>Myocardial infarction</u>**

In the event of myocardial infarction, the MB isoform (found in large quantities but not predominantly in the myocardium) rises as early as 4th hours, peaking at 24th hours.

Note: CK elevation occurs earlier than **troponin** elevation, and troponin is more specific. This is why troponin measurement is *now preferred.*

➢ **<u>Muscular diseases</u>**

In myopathies, especially **Duchenne disease**, MM CKs are highly elevated (50 to 100 times normal), but this elevation is not required for diagnosis.

In inflammatory muscular diseases such as polymyositis and dermatomyositis, CK levels are markedly increased, and can be measured to monitor progress under treatment.

29.Cholesterol

Hypercholesterolemia is a risk factor for *atherosclerosis*, as established by major epidemiological studies.
In the blood, cholesterol is carried by lipoproteins.

Low-density lipoproteins or LDLs carry 70% of total plasma cholesterol. LDL delivers cholesterol to tissues via a receptor that allows it to enter cells.

- ***values***

In adults, in the absence of other risk factors, the upper limit of normal is **5 mmol/L (2 g/L).**

<u>HDL-cholesterol</u> (is an anti-atherogenic factor)

- Male: 1 to 1.3 mmol/L (0.40 to 0.50 g/L).
- Female: 1.3 to 1.6 mmol/L (0.50 to 60 g/L).

<u>LDL-cholesterol</u>

In adults, before age 50: < 1.60 g/L (4.1 mmol/L).
Knowing that mmol/L × 0.387 = g/L.

- ***Clinical benefits***

- **<u>Hypocholesterolemia</u>**

Hypocholesterolemia is defined as a cholesterol concentration below **3.5 mmol/L**.

It is seen in ***liver failure, malabsorption and hyperthyroidism***.

Hypocholesterolemia occurs in rare familial diseases such as *Tangier disease* (accumulation of cholesterol esters in the reticuloendothelial system, tonsils or mesenteric lymph nodes), *Smith-Lemli-Opitz syndrome or SLO* (mental retardation, facial dysmorphia, genital and limb anomalies).

- **Hypercholesterolemia**

Hypercholesterolemia is defined as a cholesterol concentration above **5.5 mmol/L.**

- ***Monogenic hypercholesterolemia***

Some hypercholesterolemias - rare but the most serious - **are familial, monogenic**.

In cases of complete or partial receptor deficiency, LDL accumulates in the blood and arterial walls, leading to early hypercholesterolemia and atherosclerosis.

- ***Polygenic hypercholesterolemia***

The vast majority of hypercholesterolemias are polygenic. They do not run in families, but result from the interaction of multiple genes with environmental factors, leading to overproduction of LDL.

30.Triglyceride

Triglycerides serve as an energy reserve.

Origin: exogenous (food) and endogenous (liver synthesis). They are measured as part of the investigation of a lipid anomaly.

- ***Normal values***

Men: < 1.30 g/L (1.6 mmol/L). Women: < 1.20 g/L (1.3 mmol/L)

- ***Clinical benefits***

- **Secondary hypertriglyceridemia**

Hypertriglyceridemia of the order of 2 to 3 g/L (2.3 to 3.4 mmol/L) is common, favored *by a diet rich in sugars or alcohol. Poorly balanced diabetes, diabetic ketosis, acute alcoholism, pregnancy (where hyperestrogenism increases VLDL synthesis), nephrotic syndromes, hypothyroidism and obesity* are frequently accompanied by hypertriglyceridemia.

- **Primary hypertriglyceridemia**

Among familial primary hypertriglyceridemias, only Frederickson's type IV and IIb hyperlipoproteinemias are common.

Note: Major hypertriglyceridemia, in excess of 10 g/L (12 mmol/L) and up to 100 mmol/L, present a significant risk of acute pancreatitis and require urgent intervention.

31.Troponin

Troponins (Tn) are proteins involved in the regulation of cardiac contraction. The troponin complex comprises three proteins - T, I and C - and several isoforms.

Troponins **T (TnT) and I (TnI)** each have a cardiac isoform (TnTc and TnIc) that differs from the muscular isoforms.

Myocardial pain releases troponins into the bloodstream.

- ***Normal values***

0.04 ng/mL for TnT ;
0.1 ng/mL for TnI.

- ***Clinical benefits***

➤ **Acute coronary syndrome (ACS)**

In the event of ACS, troponins are measured as soon as possible and then every day. In the event of a negative response, a second assay is performed 6 hours later.

During myocardial ischemia, troponin T (serum or plasma) is present in the circulation.

Troponin measurement has replaced CK and other less specific markers (ASAT, LDH).

- **<u>Other cardiopulmonary conditions</u>**

Troponins rise in situations *of severe hypoxia or pulmonary hypertension.* The latest generation of "ultrasensitive" assays detect troponins in cardiac conditions other than ACS, but in a different clinical context: *myocarditis, myopericarditis, myocardiopathy, carbon monoxide intoxication, cocaine intoxication, etc.*

Troponin elevation can also be observed in *chronic renal failure and meningeal haemorrhage.*

32.Plasma ionogram

This is the measurement of the main electrolytes in plasma. electrolytes.

- ***Normal values***

Cations	mmol/L	mEq/L	Anions	mmol/L	mEq/L
Na^+	142	142	Cl^-	102	102
K^+	5	5	HCO_3^-	27	27
Ca^{++}	2,5	5	Phosphates	1	2
Mg^{++}	1	2	Protéines		16
Autres		1	Autres	4,5	8
Total		155			155

- ***Clinical benefits of some ions***

➢ **<u>Hyperkalemia (K+ > 5.3 mmol/L)</u>**

❖ ***Hyperkalemia due to reduced renal elimination***

Reduced urinary excretion of potassium is mainly due to renal insufficiency:

i. **acute** oligoanuric **renal failure** is the main cause of acute hyperkalemia.

ii. **in chronic renal failure**, hyperkalemia is moderate and delayed as long as diuresis is significant, appearing only when creatinine clearance is below 5 mL/min.

iii. **Medications**: drugs that reduce aldosterone secretion, such as ACE inhibitors, angiotensin II receptor antagonists and, to a lesser extent, non-steroidal anti-inflammatory drugs that reduce renin secretion, require kalemia monitoring in subjects at risk.

Less commonly used diuretics such as spirolactone (an aldosterone antagonist) and amiloride (which reduces tubular potassium secretion) can also cause hyperkalemia.

iv. Finally, aldosterone deficiency (Addison's disease, 21-hydroxylase deficiency) can be complicated by hyperkalemia.

❖ ***Transfer hyperkalemia***

All acidoses, whether gaseous or metabolic, can lead to hyperkalemia by transfer. In diabetic ketoacidosis, hyperkalemia is caused by acidosis, insulinopenia and hyperglycemia.

➢ **Hypokalemia (K+ < 3 mmol/L)**

Hypokalemia results *either from losses (digestive or urinary) or, more rarely, from intake deficiencies.* It is favored by alkalosis.

i. **Hypokalemia due to deficiencies or transfers**

Intake deficiencies are rarely observed except in severe alcoholics and during anorexia nervosa. Hypokalemia is rarely due to transfer (familial Westphall's periodic paralysis, hyperthyroidism periodic paralysis, chloroquine intoxication).

ii. **Hypokalemia due to digestive losses**

Digestive losses are caused by vomiting and gastric aspiration, as well as profuse diarrhea, whatever the cause - infectious, inflammatory, tumoral or drug-induced (laxative disease). Vomiting also causes alkalosis, mainly due to the loss of chlorine ion.

In case of diarrhea, acidosis due to fecal loss of bicarbonates is frequent.

In case of digestive losses, kaliuresis is low, < 10 mmol/24 h.

iii. **Hypokalemia due to urine loss**

Renal losses are due, in the majority of cases, to treatment with hypokalemic diuretics (*Esidrex*, *Fludex*, *Lasilix*), especially when prescribed to patients with secondary hyperaldosteronism.

➢ **Hyponatremia (blood sodium < 135 mmol/L)**

❖ ***Hypervolemic hyponatremia***

In this situation of significant hydrosodium inflation, with excess water greater than excess salt, blood volume is perceived as reduced by arterial baroreceptors.

Hyponatremia can occur *in heart failure, cirrhosis with ascites, nephrotic syndrome and hypoalbuminemia.* Hyponatremia is aggravated by thiazide diuretics, which alter urine dilution mechanisms and are often prescribed in these cases.

❖ ***Hypovolemic hyponatremia***

These hyponatremias are sometimes referred to as "**depletion hyponatremias**". The starting point is *extracellular dehydration*, with sodium loss proportionally greater than water loss. Hypovolemia stimulates ADH secretion.

Extracellular dehydration is manifested by tachycardia, orthostatic hypotension, skin folds, flat veins, elevated hematocrit and functional renal failure.

Hyponatremia is often associated with other electrolyte abnormalities: acidosis (diarrhea), alkalosis (vomiting), hyperkalemia (adrenal insufficiency).

- **Hypernatremia (blood sodium > 145 mmol/L)**

Hypernatremia is much **rarer** than hyponatremia. It may result from *excessive sodium intake (excessive infusion of saline, too abrupt alkalinization with sodium salt), but in common practice it is due to dehydration, i.e. water loss*

These losses can be :

- **renal** (true diabetes insipidus due to diencephalo-hypophyseal or nephrogenic lesions);
- **respiratory** (intubated, tracheotomized, travelers exposed to hot, dry atmospheres);
- **or skin (heat stroke).**

CONCLUSION

Mastering the interpretation of routine haematological and biochemical tests is an asset for every medical student in our environment.

With the advent of automated systems in our healthcare facilities, it is now possible to carry out most of these examinations automatically.

Despite this, the role of the healthcare professional remains paramount, especially as he or she is called upon to interpret the results of these examinations clinically.

From the above, we are convinced that this book will enable any student who consults it to correlate well the clinic and the results of the haematological and biochemical examinations discussed here.

As this book is not exhaustive, we suggest that you do not miss out on any future editions in this field.

References

- Réné Caquet, *250 examens de laboratoire : Prescription et intérpertation*, 11e edition, 2010, 405 pages.
- *Manuel des techniques de base pour le laboratoire médical*, based on a manual by Etienne Levy-Lambert, World Health Organization, 1982.
- epilly TROP, *Tropical Infectious Diseases*, 3e edition, 2022.

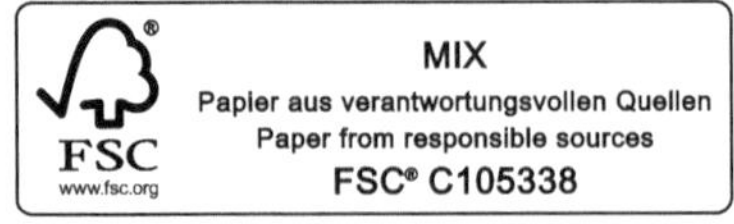

Printed by Books on Demand GmbH, Norderstedt / Germany